This Journal Belongs To:

Date: _______________

Start Weight: ___________ Current Weight:________

Weight Loss: ___________ Total Weight Loss:_____

Target Weight: _________________

Chest: _______________ Waist: _______________

Thigh: _______________ Arm: _______________

Ketone Levels:_________ Time Taken:_________

Daily Macros

Carbs: _________ Protein: _________

Fat:_____________ Calories: _________

Notes:

____

____

____

____

____

____

____

Water Intake

Exercise/Activity:

Cravings/Response:

How I'm Feeling:

Day______ Month______ Year______ | S | M | T | W | T | F | S

Breakfast

Food Item	Carbs	Fats	Proteins	Calories

Lunch

Food Item	Carbs	Fats	Proteins	Calories

Dinner

Food Item	Carbs	Fats	Proteins	Calories

Snack

Food Item	Carbs	Fats	Proteins	Calories

Totals				

Date: _______________

Start Weight: ___________ Current Weight:_________

Weight Loss: __________ Total Weight Loss:_____

Target Weight: _________________

Chest: ______________   Waist: _____________

Thigh: _____________   Arm: _______________

Ketone Levels:_________ Time Taken:__________

Daily Macros

Carbs: _________   Protein: __________

Fat:______________   Calories: __________

Notes:

____

____

____

____

____

____

____

Water Intake

Exercise/Activity:

Cravings/Response:

How I'm Feeling:

Day _____ Month _____ Year _____ | S | M | T | W | T | F | S |

Breakfast

Food Item	Carbs	Fats	Proteins	Calories

Lunch

Food Item	Carbs	Fats	Proteins	Calories

Dinner

Food Item	Carbs	Fats	Proteins	Calories

Snack

Food Item	Carbs	Fats	Proteins	Calories
Totals				

Date: _______________

Start Weight: __________ Current Weight:________

Weight Loss: __________ Total Weight Loss:______

Target Weight: ___________________

Chest: ________________ Waist: ________________

Thigh: ________________ Arm: ________________

Ketone Levels:__________ Time Taken:__________

Daily Macros

Carbs: __________ Protein: ___________

Fat:_____________ Calories: ___________

Notes:

____

____

____

____

____

____

____

 Water Intake

 Exercise/Activity:

 Cravings/Response:

 How I'm Feeling:

<u>Day</u>   <u>Month</u>   <u>Year</u> | S | M | T | W | T | F | S |

Breakfast

Food Item	Carbs	Fats	Proteins	Calories

Lunch

Food Item	Carbs	Fats	Proteins	Calories

Dinner

Food Item	Carbs	Fats	Proteins	Calories

Snack

Food Item	Carbs	Fats	Proteins	Calories
Totals				

Date: _______________

Start Weight: _____________ Current Weight:________

Weight Loss: __________ Total Weight Loss:______

Target Weight: ___________________

Chest: _______________ Waist: _______________

Thigh: _____________ Arm: _______________

Ketone Levels:__________ Time Taken:__________

Daily Macros

Carbs: __________ Protein: __________

Fat:______________ Calories: __________

Notes:

____

____

____

____

____

____

____

Water Intake

Exercise/Activity:

Cravings/Response:

How I'm Feeling:

Day _______ Month _______ Year _______ | S | M | T | W | T | F | S |

Breakfast

Food Item	Carbs	Fats	Proteins	Calories

Lunch

Food Item	Carbs	Fats	Proteins	Calories

Dinner

Food Item	Carbs	Fats	Proteins	Calories

Snack

Food Item	Carbs	Fats	Proteins	Calories
Totals				

Date: _______________

Start Weight: ___________ Current Weight:_________

Weight Loss: __________ Total Weight Loss:______

Target Weight: ____________________

Chest: ________________ Waist: ________________

Thigh: ______________ Arm: ________________

Ketone Levels:__________ Time Taken:__________

Daily Macros

Carbs: __________   Protein: ___________

Fat:________________   Calories: ___________

Notes:

____

____

____

____

____

____

____

<u>Water Intake</u>

<u>Exercise/Activity:</u>

<u>Cravings/Response:</u>

<u>How I'm Feeling:</u>

Day _______ Month _______ Year _______ | S | M | T | W | T | F | S |

Breakfast				
Food Item	Carbs	Fats	Proteins	Calories

Lunch				
Food Item	Carbs	Fats	Proteins	Calories

Dinner				
Food Item	Carbs	Fats	Proteins	Calories

Snack				
Food Item	Carbs	Fats	Proteins	Calories
Totals				

Date: _______________

Start Weight: _____________ Current Weight:__________

Weight Loss: ____________ Total Weight Loss:________

Target Weight: _________________

Chest: _______________   Waist: _______________

Thigh: _______________   Arm: _______________

Ketone Levels:__________   Time Taken:__________

Daily Macros

Carbs: __________   Protein: __________

Fat:_____________   Calories: __________

Notes:

____

____

____

____

____

____

____

 Water Intake

Exercise/Activity:

Cravings/Response:

How I'm Feeling:

Day _______ Month _______ Year _______ | S | M | T | W | T | F | S |

Breakfast

Food Item	Carbs	Fats	Proteins	Calories

Lunch

Food Item	Carbs	Fats	Proteins	Calories

Dinner

Food Item	Carbs	Fats	Proteins	Calories

Snack

Food Item	Carbs	Fats	Proteins	Calories

Totals				

Date: _______________

Start Weight: ___________ Current Weight: _______

Weight Loss: __________ Total Weight Loss: ______

Target Weight: _________________

Chest: _______________ Waist: _______________

Thigh: _______________ Arm: _______________

Ketone Levels: __________ Time Taken: __________

Daily Macros

Carbs: __________ Protein: ___________

Fat: ____________ Calories: __________

Notes:

____

____

____

____

____

____

Notes   Favorite Foods   Recipes   Meal Planning

<u>Water Intake</u>

<u>Exercise/Activity:</u>

<u>Cravings/Response:</u>

<u>How I'm Feeling:</u>

Day _______ Month _______ Year _______ | S | M | T | W | T | F | S |

Breakfast				
Food Item	Carbs	Fats	Proteins	Calories

Lunch				
Food Item	Carbs	Fats	Proteins	Calories

Dinner				
Food Item	Carbs	Fats	Proteins	Calories

Snack				
Food Item	Carbs	Fats	Proteins	Calories

Totals				

Date: _______________

Start Weight: ___________Current Weight:_________

Weight Loss: __________ Total Weight Loss:______

Target Weight: ___________________

Chest: ________________   Waist: _______________

Thigh: _______________   Arm: _______________

Ketone Levels:___________   Time Taken:__________

Daily Macros

Carbs: __________   Protein: ____________

Fat:______________   Calories: ____________

Notes:

____

____

____

____

____

____

____

Water Intake

Exercise/Activity:

Cravings/Response:

How I'm Feeling:

<u>Day</u>   <u>Month</u>   <u>Year</u>   S M T W T F S

Breakfast				
Food Item	Carbs	Fats	Proteins	Calories

Lunch				
Food Item	Carbs	Fats	Proteins	Calories

Dinner				
Food Item	Carbs	Fats	Proteins	Calories

Snack				
Food Item	Carbs	Fats	Proteins	Calories
Totals				

Date: _______________

Start Weight: ___________ Current Weight:________

Weight Loss: __________ Total Weight Loss:______

Target Weight: _________________

Chest: _______________ Waist: _______________

Thigh: _____________ Arm: _______________

Ketone Levels;__________ Time Taken:__________

Daily Macros

Carbs: _________ Protein: ___________

Fat:_____________ Calories: ___________

Notes:

____

____

____

____

____

____

____

<u>Notes   Favorite Foods   Recipes   Meal Planning</u>

<u>Water Intake</u>

<u>Exercise/Activity:</u>

<u>Cravings/Response:</u>

<u>How I'm Feeling:</u>

Day ____ Month ____ Year ____ | S | M | T | W | T | F | S |

Breakfast

Food Item	Carbs	Fats	Proteins	Calories

Lunch

Food Item	Carbs	Fats	Proteins	Calories

Dinner

Food Item	Carbs	Fats	Proteins	Calories

Snack

Food Item	Carbs	Fats	Proteins	Calories
Totals				

Date: _______________

Start Weight: ___________ Current Weight: _________

Weight Loss: ___________ Total Weight Loss: _______

Target Weight: _______________

Chest: _______________   Waist: _______________

Thigh: _______________   Arm: _______________

Ketone Levels: ___________ Time Taken: ___________

Daily Macros

Carbs: ___________   Protein: ___________

Fat: ___________   Calories: ___________

Notes:

____

____

____

____

____

____

____

 Water Intake

Exercise/Activity:

Cravings/Response:

How I'm Feeling:

Day _______ Month _______ Year _______ | S | M | T | W | T | F | S |

Breakfast

Food Item	Carbs	Fats	Proteins	Calories

Lunch

Food Item	Carbs	Fats	Proteins	Calories

Dinner

Food Item	Carbs	Fats	Proteins	Calories

Snack

Food Item	Carbs	Fats	Proteins	Calories
Totals				

Date: ______________

Start Weight: _________ Current Weight:________

Weight Loss: _________ Total Weight Loss:_____

Target Weight: __________________

Chest: ____________ Waist: ____________

Thigh: ____________ Arm: ____________

Ketone Levels:________ Time Taken:________

Daily Macros

Carbs: _________ Protein: __________

Fat:____________ Calories: __________

Notes:

____

____

____

____

____

____

____

Notes   Favorite Foods   Recipes   Meal Planning

<u>Water Intake</u>

<u>Exercise/Activity:</u>

<u>Cravings/Response:</u>

<u>How I'm Feeling:</u>

Day ______ Month ________ Year ________ | S | M | T | W | T | F | S |

Breakfast

Food Item	Carbs	Fats	Proteins	Calories

Lunch

Food Item	Carbs	Fats	Proteins	Calories

Dinner

Food Item	Carbs	Fats	Proteins	Calories

Snack

Food Item	Carbs	Fats	Proteins	Calories
Totals				

Date: _______________

Start Weight: __________ Current Weight:________

Weight Loss: __________ Total Weight Loss:______

Target Weight: ___________________

Chest: _______________ Waist: _______________

Thigh: _______________ Arm: _______________

Ketone Levels:__________ Time Taken:__________

Daily Macros

Carbs: __________ Protein: __________

Fat:______________ Calories: __________

Notes:

____

____

____

____

____

____

____

Water Intake

Exercise/Activity:

Cravings/Response:

How I'm Feeling:

Day _______ Month _______ Year _______ | S | M | T | W | T | F | S |

Breakfast

Food Item	Carbs	Fats	Proteins	Calories

Lunch

Food Item	Carbs	Fats	Proteins	Calories

Dinner

Food Item	Carbs	Fats	Proteins	Calories

Snack

Food Item	Carbs	Fats	Proteins	Calories
Totals				

Date: ______________

Start Weight: ____________ Current Weight:____________

Weight Loss: __________ Total Weight Loss:______

Target Weight: ___________________

Chest: ________________ Waist: ________________

Thigh: _______________ Arm: ________________

Ketone Levels:__________ Time Taken:__________

Daily Macros

Carbs: __________ Protein: __________

Fat:______________ Calories: __________

Notes:

____

____

____

____

____

____

Notes   Favorite Foods   Recipes   Meal Planning

 Water Intake

 Exercise/Activity:

 Cravings/Response:

 How I'm Feeling:

<u>Day</u>   <u>Month</u>   <u>Year</u> | S | M | T | W | T | F | S |

Breakfast				
Food Item	Carbs	Fats	Proteins	Calories

Lunch				
Food Item	Carbs	Fats	Proteins	Calories

Dinner				
Food Item	Carbs	Fats	Proteins	Calories

Snack				
Food Item	Carbs	Fats	Proteins	Calories
Totals				

Date: _______________

Start Weight: ____________ Current Weight:__________

Weight Loss: ____________ Total Weight Loss:______

Target Weight: _______________

Chest: _______________ Waist: _______________

Thigh: _______________ Arm: _______________

Ketone Levels:___________ Time Taken:__________

Daily Macros

Carbs: __________ Protein: ____________

Fat:____________ Calories: ____________

Notes:

____

____

____

____

____

____

____

<u>Water Intake</u>

<u>Exercise/Activity:</u>

<u>Cravings/Response:</u>

<u>How I'm Feeling:</u>

Day _______ Month _______ Year _______ | S | M | T | W | T | F | S |

Breakfast

Food Item	Carbs	Fats	Proteins	Calories

Lunch

Food Item	Carbs	Fats	Proteins	Calories

Dinner

Food Item	Carbs	Fats	Proteins	Calories

Snack

Food Item	Carbs	Fats	Proteins	Calories

Totals				

Date: ______________

Start Weight: __________ Current Weight:________

Weight Loss: _________ Total Weight Loss:______

Target Weight: _________________

Chest: ______________ Waist: _____________

Thigh: ____________ Arm: _____________

Ketone Levels:________ Time Taken:________

Daily Macros

Carbs: ________ Protein: _________

Fat:___________ Calories: __________

Notes:

____

____

____

____

____

____

Water Intake

Exercise/Activity:

Cravings/Response:

How I'm Feeling:

Day _______ Month _______ Year _______ | S | M | T | W | T | F | S |

Breakfast

Food Item	Carbs	Fats	Proteins	Calories

Lunch

Food Item	Carbs	Fats	Proteins	Calories

Dinner

Food Item	Carbs	Fats	Proteins	Calories

Snack

Food Item	Carbs	Fats	Proteins	Calories
Totals				

Date: ______________

Start Weight: __________ Current Weight:________

Weight Loss: __________ Total Weight Loss:______

Target Weight: _________________

Chest: ______________ Waist: ______________

Thigh: ______________ Arm: ______________

Ketone Levels:__________ Time Taken:__________

Daily Macros

Carbs: __________ Protein: __________

Fat:______________ Calories: __________

Notes:

____

____

____

____

____

____

____

 Water Intake

Exercise/Activity:

Cravings/Response:

How I'm Feeling:

<u>Day</u>   <u>Month</u>   <u>Year</u>   S M T W T F S

Breakfast

Food Item	Carbs	Fats	Proteins	Calories

Lunch

Food Item	Carbs	Fats	Proteins	Calories

Dinner

Food Item	Carbs	Fats	Proteins	Calories

Snack

Food Item	Carbs	Fats	Proteins	Calories
Totals				

Date: _______________

Start Weight: _____________ Current Weight:_________

Weight Loss: __________ Total Weight Loss:______

Target Weight: ____________________

Chest: _______________   Waist: _______________

Thigh: _______________   Arm: _______________

Ketone Levels:__________   Time Taken:__________

Daily Macros

Carbs: __________   Protein: ____________

Fat:______________   Calories: ____________

Notes:

____

____

____

____

____

____

____

<u>Water Intake</u>

<u>Exercise/Activity:</u>

<u>Cravings/Response:</u>

<u>How I'm Feeling:</u>

<u>Day</u>   <u>Month</u>   <u>Year</u> | S | M | T | W | T | F | S |

Breakfast

Food Item	Carbs	Fats	Proteins	Calories

Lunch

Food Item	Carbs	Fats	Proteins	Calories

Dinner

Food Item	Carbs	Fats	Proteins	Calories

Snack

Food Item	Carbs	Fats	Proteins	Calories
Totals				

Date: ______________

Start Weight: ___________ Current Weight:________

Weight Loss: __________ Total Weight Loss:_____

Target Weight: ___________________

Chest: _______________ Waist: _______________

Thigh: ______________ Arm: _______________

Ketone Levels:__________ Time Taken:__________

Daily Macros

Carbs: __________   Protein: ___________

Fat:_____________   Calories: ___________

Notes:

____

____

____

____

____

____

____

<u>Water Intake</u>

<u>Exercise/Activity:</u>

<u>Cravings/Response:</u>

<u>How I'm Feeling:</u>

Day _______ Month _______ Year _______ | S | M | T | W | T | F | S |

Breakfast

Food Item	Carbs	Fats	Proteins	Calories

Lunch

Food Item	Carbs	Fats	Proteins	Calories

Dinner

Food Item	Carbs	Fats	Proteins	Calories

Snack

Food Item	Carbs	Fats	Proteins	Calories
Totals				

Date: _______________

Start Weight: _______________ Current Weight:_______________

Weight Loss: _______________ Total Weight Loss:_______________

Target Weight: _______________

Chest: _______________ Waist: _______________

Thigh: _______________ Arm: _______________

Ketone Levels:_______________ Time Taken:_______________

Daily Macros

Carbs: _______________ Protein: _______________

Fat:_______________ Calories: _______________

Notes:

____

____

____

____

____

____

____

Water Intake

Exercise/Activity:

Cravings/Response:

How I'm Feeling:

<u>Day</u>   <u>Month</u>   <u>Year</u> | S | M | T | W | T | F | S |

Breakfast				
Food Item	Carbs	Fats	Proteins	Calories

Lunch				
Food Item	Carbs	Fats	Proteins	Calories

Dinner				
Food Item	Carbs	Fats	Proteins	Calories

Snack				
Food Item	Carbs	Fats	Proteins	Calories

Totals	Carbs	Fats	Proteins	Calories

Date: _______________

Start Weight: _____________ Current Weight:_________

Weight Loss: ___________ Total Weight Loss:______

Target Weight: _________________

Chest: ________________   Waist: ________________

Thigh: ________________   Arm: _________________

Ketone Levels:___________ Time Taken:___________

Daily Macros

Carbs: ___________   Protein: ____________

Fat:_____________   Calories: ____________

Notes:

____

____

____

____

____

____

____

Notes   Favorite Foods   Recipes   Meal Planning

Water Intake

Exercise/Activity:

Cravings/Response:

How I'm Feeling:

Day ______ Month ______ Year ______ | S | M | T | W | T | F | S |

Breakfast

Food Item	Carbs	Fats	Proteins	Calories

Lunch

Food Item	Carbs	Fats	Proteins	Calories

Dinner

Food Item	Carbs	Fats	Proteins	Calories

Snack

Food Item	Carbs	Fats	Proteins	Calories
Totals				

Date: _______________

Start Weight: _____________ Current Weight:_________

Weight Loss: ___________ Total Weight Loss:______

Target Weight: ______________________

Chest: ________________ Waist: ________________

Thigh: ________________ Arm: _________________

Ketone Levels:____________ Time Taken:___________

Daily Macros

Carbs: ____________ Protein: ____________

Fat:______________ Calories: ____________

Notes:

____

____

____

____

____

____

____

Notes   Favorite Foods   Recipes   Meal Planning

 Water Intake

Exercise/Activity:

Cravings/Response:

How I'm Feeling:

Day   Month   Year | S | M | T | W | T | F | S |

Breakfast

Food Item	Carbs	Fats	Proteins	Calories

Lunch

Food Item	Carbs	Fats	Proteins	Calories

Dinner

Food Item	Carbs	Fats	Proteins	Calories

Snack

Food Item	Carbs	Fats	Proteins	Calories
Totals				

Date: _______________

Start Weight: __________ Current Weight:_______

Weight Loss: __________ Total Weight Loss:______

Target Weight: _________________

Chest: _______________ Waist: _______________

Thigh: _______________ Arm: _______________

Ketone Levels;_________ Time Taken:_________

Daily Macros

Carbs: _________ Protein: _________

Fat:_____________ Calories: _________

Notes:

____

____

____

____

____

____

____

<u>Notes   Favorite Foods   Recipes   Meal Planning</u>

Water Intake

Exercise/Activity:

Cravings/Response:

How I'm Feeling:

Day _______ Month _______ Year _______ | S | M | T | W | T | F | S |

Breakfast

Food Item	Carbs	Fats	Proteins	Calories

Lunch

Food Item	Carbs	Fats	Proteins	Calories

Dinner

Food Item	Carbs	Fats	Proteins	Calories

Snack

Food Item	Carbs	Fats	Proteins	Calories
Totals				

Date: ___________________

Start Weight: _____________ Current Weight:___________

Weight Loss: _____________ Total Weight Loss:_________

Target Weight: _________________________

Chest: _______________ Waist: _______________

Thigh: _______________ Arm: _______________

Ketone Levels:___________ Time Taken:___________

Daily Macros

Carbs: _____________ Protein: _______________

Fat:_______________ Calories: _______________

Notes:

____

____

____

____

____

____

____

 Water Intake

 Exercise/Activity:

 Cravings/Response:

 How I'm Feeling:

Day _______ Month _______ Year _______ | S | M | T | W | T | F | S |

Breakfast

Food Item	Carbs	Fats	Proteins	Calories

Lunch

Food Item	Carbs	Fats	Proteins	Calories

Dinner

Food Item	Carbs	Fats	Proteins	Calories

Snack

Food Item	Carbs	Fats	Proteins	Calories
Totals				

Date: ___________________

Start Weight: ______________ Current Weight:__________

Weight Loss: ____________ Total Weight Loss:______

Target Weight: ___________________

Chest: ________________ Waist: ________________

Thigh: ________________ Arm: ________________

Ketone Levels:__________ Time Taken:__________

Daily Macros

Carbs: ____________ Protein: ______________

Fat:______________ Calories: ____________

Notes:

____

____

____

____

____

____

____

 Water Intake

Exercise/Activity:

Cravings/Response:

How I'm Feeling:

Day _______ Month _______ Year _______ | S | M | T | W | T | F | S |

Breakfast

Food Item	Carbs	Fats	Proteins	Calories

Lunch

Food Item	Carbs	Fats	Proteins	Calories

Dinner

Food Item	Carbs	Fats	Proteins	Calories

Snack

Food Item	Carbs	Fats	Proteins	Calories
Totals				

Date: _______________

Start Weight: ___________ Current Weight:_________

Weight Loss: ___________ Total Weight Loss:______

Target Weight: _________________

Chest: _______________ Waist: _______________

Thigh: _______________ Arm: _______________

Ketone Levels:_________ Time Taken:__________

Daily Macros

Carbs: __________ Protein: ___________

Fat:_____________ Calories: ___________

Notes:

____

____

____

____

____

____

____

Notes   Favorite Foods   Recipes   Meal Planning

Water Intake

Exercise/Activity:

Cravings/Response:

How I'm Feeling:

<u>Day</u>   <u>Month</u>   <u>Year</u> | S | M | T | W | T | F | S |

Breakfast

Food Item	Carbs	Fats	Proteins	Calories

Lunch

Food Item	Carbs	Fats	Proteins	Calories

Dinner

Food Item	Carbs	Fats	Proteins	Calories

Snack

Food Item	Carbs	Fats	Proteins	Calories
Totals				

Date: _______________

Start Weight: _____________ Current Weight:_________

Weight Loss: ___________ Total Weight Loss:_____

Target Weight: ____________________

Chest: _______________ Waist: ______________

Thigh: _______________ Arm: ________________

Ketone Levels:__________ Time Taken:_________

Daily Macros

Carbs: __________ Protein: ___________

Fat:_______________ Calories: ___________

Notes:

____

____

____

____

____

____

____

<u>Water Intake</u>

<u>Exercise/Activity:</u>

<u>Cravings/Response:</u>

<u>How I'm Feeling:</u>

Day______ Month______ Year______ | S | M | T | W | T | F | S |

Breakfast

Food Item	Carbs	Fats	Proteins	Calories

Lunch

Food Item	Carbs	Fats	Proteins	Calories

Dinner

Food Item	Carbs	Fats	Proteins	Calories

Snack

Food Item	Carbs	Fats	Proteins	Calories
Totals				

Date: _______________

Start Weight: ____________ Current Weight:__________

Weight Loss: ___________ Total Weight Loss:______

Target Weight: _______________

Chest: _______________ Waist: _______________

Thigh: _______________ Arm: _______________

Ketone Levels:__________ Time Taken:__________

Daily Macros

Carbs: ___________ Protein: ___________

Fat:_____________ Calories: ___________

Notes:

____

____

____

____

____

____

Water Intake

Exercise/Activity:

Cravings/Response:

How I'm Feeling:

Day   Month   Year   S | M | T | W | T | F | S

Breakfast

Food Item	Carbs	Fats	Proteins	Calories

Lunch

Food Item	Carbs	Fats	Proteins	Calories

Dinner

Food Item	Carbs	Fats	Proteins	Calories

Snack

Food Item	Carbs	Fats	Proteins	Calories
Totals				

Date: _______________

Start Weight: ___________ Current Weight:_________

Weight Loss: __________ Total Weight Loss:______

Target Weight: ___________________

Chest: ______________ Waist: ______________

Thigh: ______________ Arm: ______________

Ketone Levels:__________ Time Taken:__________

Daily Macros

Carbs: __________ Protein: ___________

Fat:_____________ Calories: __________

Notes:

____

____

____

____

____

____

____

Notes   Favorite Foods   Recipes   Meal Planning

Water Intake

Exercise/Activity:

Cravings/Response:

How I'm Feeling:

Breakfast

Food Item	Carbs	Fats	Proteins	Calories

Lunch

Food Item	Carbs	Fats	Proteins	Calories

Dinner

Food Item	Carbs	Fats	Proteins	Calories

Snack

Food Item	Carbs	Fats	Proteins	Calories
Totals				

Date: _______________

Start Weight: __________ Current Weight:_________

Weight Loss: __________ Total Weight Loss:______

Target Weight: _________________

Chest: _____________   Waist: _____________

Thigh: _____________   Arm: _______________

Ketone Levels:_________   Time Taken:_________

Daily Macros

Carbs: _________   Protein: __________

Fat:____________   Calories: __________

Notes:

____

____

____

____

____

____

____

Water Intake

Exercise/Activity:

Cravings/Response:

How I'm Feeling:

Day _______ Month _______ Year _______ | S | M | T | W | T | F | S |

Breakfast				
Food Item	Carbs	Fats	Proteins	Calories

Lunch				
Food Item	Carbs	Fats	Proteins	Calories

Dinner				
Food Item	Carbs	Fats	Proteins	Calories

Snack				
Food Item	Carbs	Fats	Proteins	Calories
Totals				

Date: _______________

Start Weight: _____________ Current Weight:__________

Weight Loss: ____________ Total Weight Loss:______

Target Weight: ________________________

Chest: __________________ Waist: __________________

Thigh: __________________ Arm: ___________________

Ketone Levels:____________ Time Taken:____________

Daily Macros

Carbs: ______________ Protein: ______________

Fat:________________ Calories: ______________

Notes:

____

____

____

____

____

____

Water Intake

Exercise/Activity:

Cravings/Response:

How I'm Feeling:

| Day | Month | Year | | S | M | T | W | T | F | S |

Breakfast				
Food Item	Carbs	Fats	Proteins	Calories

Lunch				
Food Item	Carbs	Fats	Proteins	Calories

Dinner				
Food Item	Carbs	Fats	Proteins	Calories

Snack				
Food Item	Carbs	Fats	Proteins	Calories
Totals				

Date: _______________

Start Weight: _____________ Current Weight:_________

Weight Loss: ___________ Total Weight Loss:______

Target Weight: ___________________

Chest: _______________   Waist: _______________

Thigh: _______________   Arm: _______________

Ketone Levels:__________   Time Taken:__________

Daily Macros

Carbs: __________   Protein: ___________

Fat:_______________   Calories: __________

Notes:

____

____

____

____

____

____

____

Water Intake

Exercise/Activity:

Cravings/Response:

How I'm Feeling:

Day _______ Month _______ Year _______ | S | M | T | W | T | F | S |

Breakfast

Food Item	Carbs	Fats	Proteins	Calories

Lunch

Food Item	Carbs	Fats	Proteins	Calories

Dinner

Food Item	Carbs	Fats	Proteins	Calories

Snack

Food Item	Carbs	Fats	Proteins	Calories

Totals				

Date: _______________

Start Weight: __________ Current Weight:________

Weight Loss: __________ Total Weight Loss:______

Target Weight: ____________________

Chest: ______________ Waist: ______________

Thigh: ______________ Arm: ______________

Ketone Levels:__________ Time Taken:__________

Daily Macros

Carbs: __________ Protein: __________

Fat:______________ Calories: __________

Notes:

____

____

____

____

____

____

____

<u>Notes   Favorite Foods   Recipes   Meal Planning</u>

<u>Water Intake</u>

<u>Exercise/Activity:</u>

<u>Cravings/Response:</u>

<u>How I'm Feeling:</u>

Day _______ Month _______ Year _______ | S | M | T | W | T | F | S |

Breakfast

Food Item	Carbs	Fats	Proteins	Calories

Lunch

Food Item	Carbs	Fats	Proteins	Calories

Dinner

Food Item	Carbs	Fats	Proteins	Calories

Snack

Food Item	Carbs	Fats	Proteins	Calories
Totals				

Date: ___________________

Start Weight: _____________ Current Weight:___________

Weight Loss: ____________ Total Weight Loss:_______

Target Weight: __________________

Chest: ________________   Waist: ________________

Thigh: ______________   Arm: ________________

Ketone Levels:___________   Time Taken:____________

Daily Macros

Carbs: __________   Protein: ____________

Fat:________________   Calories: ___________

Notes:

____

____

____

____

____

____

____

 Water Intake

Exercise/Activity:

Cravings/Response:

How I'm Feeling:

Day _______ Month _______ Year _______ | S | M | T | W | T | F | S |

Breakfast

Food Item	Carbs	Fats	Proteins	Calories

Lunch

Food Item	Carbs	Fats	Proteins	Calories

Dinner

Food Item	Carbs	Fats	Proteins	Calories

Snack

Food Item	Carbs	Fats	Proteins	Calories
Totals				

Date: _________________

Start Weight: ____________ Current Weight:__________

Weight Loss: ___________ Total Weight Loss:______

Target Weight: __________________

Chest: ________________ Waist: ________________

Thigh: ______________ Arm: ________________

Ketone Levels:__________ Time Taken:_________

Daily Macros

Carbs: __________ Protein: ___________

Fat:_____________ Calories: __________

Notes:

____

____

____

____

____

____

____

Water Intake

Exercise/Activity:

Cravings/Response:

How I'm Feeling:

<u>Day</u>   <u>Month</u>   <u>Year</u> | S | M | T | W | T | F | S |

Breakfast

Food Item	Carbs	Fats	Proteins	Calories

Lunch

Food Item	Carbs	Fats	Proteins	Calories

Dinner

Food Item	Carbs	Fats	Proteins	Calories

Snack

Food Item	Carbs	Fats	Proteins	Calories
Totals				

Date: _______________

Start Weight: __________ Current Weight:_________

Weight Loss: __________ Total Weight Loss:______

Target Weight: _____________________

Chest: _______________ Waist: _______________

Thigh: _______________ Arm: _______________

Ketone Levels:_________ Time Taken:__________

Daily Macros

Carbs: __________ Protein: ___________

Fat:_____________ Calories: ___________

Notes:

____

____

____

____

____

____

____

<u>Notes   Favorite Foods   Recipes   Meal Planning</u>

 Water Intake

Exercise/Activity:

Cravings/Response:

How I'm Feeling:

Day _______ Month _______ Year _______ | S | M | T | W | T | F | S |

Breakfast

Food Item	Carbs	Fats	Proteins	Calories

Lunch

Food Item	Carbs	Fats	Proteins	Calories

Dinner

Food Item	Carbs	Fats	Proteins	Calories

Snack

Food Item	Carbs	Fats	Proteins	Calories
Totals				

Date: ______________

Start Weight: __________ Current Weight:________

Weight Loss: __________ Total Weight Loss:______

Target Weight: ____________________

Chest: ______________   Waist: ______________

Thigh: ______________   Arm: ______________

Ketone Levels: ________   Time Taken: ________

Daily Macros

Carbs: __________   Protein: __________

Fat: ____________   Calories: __________

Notes:

____

____

____

____

____

____

Notes   Favorite Foods   Recipes   Meal Planning

 Water Intake

 Exercise/Activity:

 Cravings/Response:

 How I'm Feeling:

Day _______ Month _______ Year _______ | S | M | T | W | T | F | S |

Breakfast

Food Item	Carbs	Fats	Proteins	Calories

Lunch

Food Item	Carbs	Fats	Proteins	Calories

Dinner

Food Item	Carbs	Fats	Proteins	Calories

Snack

Food Item	Carbs	Fats	Proteins	Calories
Totals				

Date: _______________

Start Weight: ___________ Current Weight:__________

Weight Loss: ___________ Total Weight Loss:_______

Target Weight: _______________________

Chest: _______________ Waist: _______________

Thigh: _______________ Arm: _______________

Ketone Levels:___________ Time Taken:___________

Daily Macros

Carbs: ___________ Protein: ___________

Fat:___________ Calories: ___________

Notes:

____

____

____

____

____

____

____

Notes Favorite Foods Recipes Meal Planning

 Water Intake

Exercise/Activity:

Cravings/Response:

How I'm Feeling:

<u>Day</u> <u>Month</u> <u>Year</u> | S | M | T | W | T | F | S |

Breakfast

Food Item	Carbs	Fats	Proteins	Calories

Lunch

Food Item	Carbs	Fats	Proteins	Calories

Dinner

Food Item	Carbs	Fats	Proteins	Calories

Snack

Food Item	Carbs	Fats	Proteins	Calories
Totals				

Date: _______________

Start Weight: __________ Current Weight:________

Weight Loss: __________ Total Weight Loss:_____

Target Weight: ___________________

Chest: _______________ Waist: _______________

Thigh: _______________ Arm: _______________

Ketone Levels:__________ Time Taken:__________

Daily Macros

Carbs: __________ Protein: ___________

Fat:_____________ Calories: ___________

Notes:

____

____

____

____

____

____

<u>Water Intake</u>

<u>Exercise/Activity:</u>

<u>Cravings/Response:</u>

<u>How I'm Feeling:</u>

<u>Day</u>   <u>Month</u>   <u>Year</u> | S | M | T | W | T | F | S |

Breakfast				
Food Item	Carbs	Fats	Proteins	Calories

Lunch				
Food Item	Carbs	Fats	Proteins	Calories

Dinner				
Food Item	Carbs	Fats	Proteins	Calories

Snack				
Food Item	Carbs	Fats	Proteins	Calories
Totals				

Date: _______________

Start Weight: ___________ Current Weight:_________

Weight Loss: __________ Total Weight Loss:_______

Target Weight: _________________

Chest: _____________ Waist: _____________

Thigh: _____________ Arm: _____________

Ketone Levels:_________ Time Taken:__________

Daily Macros

Carbs: __________ Protein: ___________

Fat:____________ Calories: ___________

Notes:

____

____

____

____

____

____

____

 Water Intake

Exercise/Activity:

Cravings/Response:

How I'm Feeling:

Day _______ Month _______ Year _______ S M T W T F S

Breakfast

Food Item	Carbs	Fats	Proteins	Calories

Lunch

Food Item	Carbs	Fats	Proteins	Calories

Dinner

Food Item	Carbs	Fats	Proteins	Calories

Snack

Food Item	Carbs	Fats	Proteins	Calories
Totals				

Date: _______________

Start Weight: __________ Current Weight:________

Weight Loss: __________ Total Weight Loss:______

Target Weight: ____________________

Chest: ______________ Waist: ______________

Thigh: ______________ Arm: ______________

Ketone Levels:__________ Time Taken: __________

Daily Macros

Carbs: __________ Protein: __________

Fat:______________ Calories: __________

Notes:

____

____

____

____

____

____

____

 Water Intake

Exercise/Activity:

Cravings/Response:

How I'm Feeling:

<u>Day</u>   <u>Month</u>   <u>Year</u> | S | M | T | W | T | F | S |

Breakfast				
Food Item	Carbs	Fats	Proteins	Calories

Lunch				
Food Item	Carbs	Fats	Proteins	Calories

Dinner				
Food Item	Carbs	Fats	Proteins	Calories

Food Item	Snack			
	Carbs	Fats	Proteins	Calories
Totals				

Date: _______________

Start Weight: _____________ Current Weight:__________

Weight Loss: ___________ Total Weight Loss:________

Target Weight: _________________

Chest: _______________ Waist: _______________

Thigh: _______________ Arm: _______________

Ketone Levels:__________ Time Taken:__________

Daily Macros

Carbs: __________ Protein: ___________

Fat:_____________ Calories: ___________

Notes:

____

____

____

____

____

____

____

<u>Water Intake</u>

<u>Exercise/Activity:</u>

<u>Cravings/Response:</u>

<u>How I'm Feeling:</u>

<u>Day</u>　　　<u>Month</u>　　　<u>Year</u>　　　　| S | M | T | W | T | F | S |

Breakfast

Food Item	Carbs	Fats	Proteins	Calories

Lunch

Food Item	Carbs	Fats	Proteins	Calories

Dinner

Food Item	Carbs	Fats	Proteins	Calories

Snack

Food Item	Carbs	Fats	Proteins	Calories
Totals				

Date: __________________

Start Weight: _____________ Current Weight: _________

Weight Loss: ___________ Total Weight Loss: _______

Target Weight: __________________

Chest: ________________   Waist: _______________

Thigh: _____________   Arm: ________________

Ketone Levels: __________   Time Taken: __________

Daily Macros

Carbs: __________   Protein: ___________

Fat: _____________   Calories: ___________

Notes:

____

____

____

____

____

____

Notes   Favorite Foods   Recipes   Meal Planning

 Water Intake

Exercise/Activity:

Cravings/Response:

How I'm Feeling:

Day _______ Month _______ Year _______ | S | M | T | W | T | F | S |

Breakfast

Food Item	Carbs	Fats	Proteins	Calories

Lunch

Food Item	Carbs	Fats	Proteins	Calories

Dinner

Food Item	Carbs	Fats	Proteins	Calories

Snack

Food Item	Carbs	Fats	Proteins	Calories
Totals				

Date: _______________

Start Weight: ___________ Current Weight:_________

Weight Loss: __________ Total Weight Loss:_______

Target Weight: _________________

Chest: _______________ Waist: _______________

Thigh: _____________ Arm: _______________

Ketone Levels:_________ Time Taken:__________

Daily Macros

Carbs: _________ Protein: __________

Fat:____________ Calories: __________

Notes:

____

____

____

____

____

____

____

<u>Water Intake</u>

<u>Exercise/Activity:</u>

<u>Cravings/Response:</u>

<u>How I'm Feeling:</u>

<u>Day</u>   <u>Month</u>   <u>Year</u> | S | M | T | W | T | F | S |

Breakfast				
Food Item	Carbs	Fats	Proteins	Calories

Lunch				
Food Item	Carbs	Fats	Proteins	Calories

Dinner				
Food Item	Carbs	Fats	Proteins	Calories

Snack				
Food Item	Carbs	Fats	Proteins	Calories
Totals				

Date: _______________

Start Weight: ___________Current Weight:_________

Weight Loss: ___________ Total Weight Loss:______

Target Weight: _________________

Chest: _______________   Waist: _______________

Thigh: _______________   Arm: _______________

Ketone Levels:_________   Time Taken:_________

Daily Macros

Carbs: __________   Protein: ___________

Fat:_____________   Calories: ___________

Notes:

____

____

____

____

____

____

____

 Water Intake

Exercise/Activity:

Cravings/Response:

How I'm Feeling:

<u>Day</u>   <u>Month</u>   <u>Year</u> | S | M | T | W | T | F | S |

Breakfast

Food Item	Carbs	Fats	Proteins	Calories

Lunch

Food Item	Carbs	Fats	Proteins	Calories

Dinner

Food Item	Carbs	Fats	Proteins	Calories

Snack

Food Item	Carbs	Fats	Proteins	Calories
Totals				

Date: _______________

Start Weight: ___________ Current Weight:________

Weight Loss: __________ Total Weight Loss:______

Target Weight: ___________________

Chest: ______________ Waist: ______________

Thigh: ______________ Arm: ______________

Ketone Levels:__________ Time Taken:__________

Daily Macros

Carbs: __________ Protein: __________

Fat:____________ Calories: __________

Notes:

____

____

____

____

____

____

____

 Water Intake

Exercise/Activity:

Cravings/Response:

How I'm Feeling:

Day   Month   Year ____ $\boxed{S}$ $\boxed{M}$ $\boxed{T}$ $\boxed{W}$ $\boxed{T}$ $\boxed{F}$ $\boxed{S}$

Breakfast

Food Item	Carbs	Fats	Proteins	Calories

Lunch

Food Item	Carbs	Fats	Proteins	Calories

Dinner

Food Item	Carbs	Fats	Proteins	Calories

Snack

Food Item	Carbs	Fats	Proteins	Calories
Totals				

9 781726 867740